Introduction

This book is mainly focused on World health organization's two important and interlinked concepts, health for all and primary health care. Both are very important regarding the wellbeing of world population and both are related to each other very closely. Immunization against infectious diseases is also a very important segment in primary health care. It is also discussed here. Apart from that, a brief discussion done about other effective medicine practicing methods, such as Ayurveda, acupuncture and homeopathy. The important factor which is equally related to all three above methods is that all these are still in practice and developing and still effective regarding people's well-being.

All these fields are vast and important. What done here is discussing them briefly and study them to gain knowledge to expand the knowledge base; so can be used in the future in nursing practice. To realize that many practices a nurse do during the working hours, actually related to these major concepts and programs is also a major advantage of this particular assessment. So the using of these concepts in future nursing practices can be done even more effectively as the purpose and importance are known. Actually the foundation of effective nursing practice is based on primary health care. By going through this assessment one can realize that it is true.

Health for all

Health for all is an important goal of world health organization since 1970. The WHO targeted to reach health for all in year 2000. It is used as the base strategy of their primary health care programs to promote health and to enhance the quality of life and human dignity of the people all around the world. The final expected result is securing the health and well-being of world population.

WHO expected to develop a health system in which health facilities are within reach of anybody. But this doesn't just mean that the availability of health services or hospitals; but enabling socially and economically productive life for every person in any given society. The basic effort is to eliminate all the resistances against wellbeing of people; including malnutrition, ignorance, contaminated drinking water, unhygienic housing, lack of doctors and other medical staff, hospital beds and drugs and vaccines and etc.

W.H.O. said that health is a major objective of economic development of a country. Educating people about the health and how to reach optimum level of health is a must. To reach the state of health for all, as much as medical care department of a society try, other departments such as agriculture, industry, education and communication branches of that society should get together and try.

Medical care and also public health are equally important in this particular concept. In every village basic medical help should be within reach and it should be backed up by more advanced and specialized medical care. The other important aspect is immunization program. It should also be globalized and provide universal coverage.

To achieve this goal "health for all", governments of countries have a major role to play. They should adopt the concept to the health systems of their countries and apply it with the desire of giving higher quality of life to their citizens.

Two decades later, WHO Director General Lee Jong-wook (2003–2006) reaffirmed the concept in the World Health Report 2003.

 "Health for all became the slogan for a movement. It was not just an ideal but an organizing principle: everybody needs and is entitled to the highest possible standard of health. The principles remain indispensable for a coherent vision of global health. Turning that vision into reality calls for clarity both on the possibilities and on the obstacles that have slowed and in some cases reversed progress towards meeting the health needs of all people. We have a real opportunity now to make progress that will mean longer, healthier lives for millions of people, turn despair into realistic hope, and lay the foundations for improved health for generations to come."

Sri Lanka too has driven there strategies in primary health care sector to achieve the goal of health for all concept. Our country has implied many programs with help of WHO and actually gained a rapid development in primary health care.

Primary health care

Primary health care means essential health care to provide better health for all. It is based on practical, scientifically sound and socially acceptable methods and technology. It should be universally accessible to individuals and families in the community through their full participation. And the cost should be affordable in every stage. WHO introduced this concept in 1978 on a conference held at Alma Ata. WHO also published "Alma Ata declaration" based on this conference and it became the core concept for the reaching of goal of health for all. The core objective of the whole process is to build self-reliance and self-determination of the people around the globe.

W.H.O believe that by reducing exclusion and social disparities in health, organizing health services around people's needs and expectations, integrating health into all sectors, pursuing collaborative models of policy dialogue and increasing stakeholder participation they can achieve this goal.

Alma Ata declaration has some important principles. These should be included in national policies of health in order to provide better care for all with the coordination with other sectors.

Equitable distribution of health care - Irrespective of once gender, age, caste, color, urban/rural location and social class, one should be able to gain access to primary care and other health services.

Community participation – To gain the fullest use of all the available resources, community participation is important.

Health workforce development –To provide an effective health care the health team should be stronger. It requires trained physicians, nurses and other health care associated professionals.

Use of appropriate technology –To provide health care most effectively using of latest and appropriate technologies is necessary

Multi-sectional approach –To improve the health of a country, sectors such as agriculture, education, communication, housing, public workers, rural development, industry and community organization

A basic concept of public health is that every individual who is protected from a disease as a result of an immunization is one less individual capable of transmitting the disease to others. Individuals who have been immunized serve as a protective barrier for other individuals who have not been immunized.

Immunization against infectious was intodused to the sri lanka health system in 19th centuary. It has been very successful since then and is now covering vast number of diseases. The main target is to immunize children against such diseases and to reduce the spread of such disesases and to eliminate such diseases from the world.

In 1886 a vaccine against smallfox was intrdused. It was a great success and smallfox was totally eliminate from the country and the globe with the use of this vaccine. And this same result is expected the same result with poliomyelitis.

Expand program on ommunization (EPI) is the most important program against infectious diseases. It is a joint venture of WHO (World Health Organization) and UNICEF (the United Nation's Children's Fund). It was intrdused in 1978. It is a great success in Sri Lanka's health system. With the help of this programme Sri lanka has successfully immunized children against infectious diseases, around the whole country.Actually Immunizing a child not only protects that child but also other children by increasing the general level of immunity and minimising the spread of infection.

EPI was introduced with the hope to control childhood T.B., tetanus, whooping cough, diphtheria, polio and neo-natal tetanus. In 1988 the main focus was changed from controlling diseases to eliminating them. In later years vaccine against Rubella, Hepatitis B introduced. This vaccine is called Pentavelant. (Japanese Encephalitis) JE vaccine was introduced in 1987 for the high risk areas.

Immunity is devided into two major components. Those are non specific immunity and specific immunity.

The body has ability to tolerate materials indigenious to it and eliminate materials forign to it.By identifying harmful substances to body which are called antigens, the immune system of the body attack them using antibodies. This process is called specific immunity.This too has two major components. Those are active immunity nad passive immunity.

Active immunity is provided by a person's own immune system. This type of immunity can come from exposure to a disease or from vaccination. And this type of immunity usually long last or permanent.

Passive immunity means transfers of antibodies from immune to nun- immune person. It is usually happens from mother to child through placenta. And in some diseases transferring of antibodies done artificially as a vaccine. E.g.:- tetanus. But this kind of protection is usually short lived.

Traditional Indigenous system of medicine in Sri Lanka

Sri Lanka has a traditional medicine system which about three thousand years old. It is based on system called "desiya chikithsa".It was also influenced by Indian traditional medicine methods and some Arab methods. This system is usually called "Ayurvedha". The ayurvedic system is mostly based on ancient prescriptions handed down from generations to generations. But there are some important references in written which are in use even now a days. "Sarartha Sangrahaya" which was written by King Buddadasa – one of most famous ancient aurvedic doctor- is one of them.

The aurvedic system is closely related with nature and Buddhism. All the ingredients using in treatment are natural elements from surrounding, Just as the modern medicine is based on physics, Chemistry, Botany, and Zoology. Ayurveda is based on Indian or Hindu Philosophy. The theory of macrocosm and microcosm. It believes that the matter is composed of five elements (Panchamaha buta).They are Prithvi (earth or hardness), APO (water or liquid), Theja (fire or energy), Vayu (gases state of matter) . All the diseases are because unbalancing of these five elements. Treatment is to reverse whatever unbalanced.

Development of Acupuncture

The meaning of acupuncture is needle puncture. This is a system developed in ancient China. The very first clue about acupuncture is from around 2600BC. Acupuncture believes that to a certain disease a certain area of the skin shows more sensitive. And there are certain areas representing certain body organs. Depending on this concept the treatment methods are developed.

Qi, "the energy" is the major concept in acupuncture. "The spots", sensitive areas described above are connected to each other via lines. So the energy flows from one another through lines. According to acupuncture a certain amount of energy is given on once birth. Illness means imbalance of this energy in various points.

By the use of needle acupuncture affect the energy level of organs which leads to stimulate or reduse of that particular organ's action. That way can use to pain control, stress relief, and for many other physical diseases. From china acupuncture travelled to Europe in seventeenth century. Around 1940 acupuncture was gaining attention of western physicians regarding pain relief. Books were also published explaining the methods of acupuncture from around this time.

.

Acupuncture is now well accepted method in western medicine. The method is widely use in pain control and stress management. In some countries, for some operations, instead of anesthesia, physicians use acupuncture methods. So the organs of the patient are not affected by artificial anesthetic agents. Apart from that, acupuncture is in a stage of expanding. Chinese are developing new methods based on ancient texts.

Homeopathy

The major concept in homeopathy is law of similes or "like cures like" as it called. It says that when a substance in large doses causes certain symptoms, in small doses it can cure these same symptoms. Homeopathy uses many natural ingredients to produce remedies such as herbs, minerals, various plants, snake venom and etc.

Homeopathy believes every physical illness has mental and emotional components. So the remedy is made considering all three components together. The aim on the remedy is to stimulate the body's own healing mechanism. To do they need to consider of all three above components together.

Usually homeopathy does not have any side effects. It is one of the major concerns for people to take homeopathy treatment instead of western medicine. Actually in many countries homeopathy has schools and recognized by the governments as a legal method to practice. Homeopathy practitioners are now even has expanded there treatments towards diseases like AIDS and cancers.

What can a nurse do to make health for all a reality.
Health For All depends on continued progress in medical care and public health.In both these sectors nurses are playing a vital role. Medical care is usually done when a person is hospitalized and from the admission to

the discharge nurses are intervincing in every step. In these step a nurse can provide various services to the patient to prevent him/her from many diseases. Health education is one of such important intervince, As the nurse knows the general condition of the patient the nurse can organize the facts to educate the patient about his/her wellbeing in the future. If the patient has any particular disease , nurse can educate the patient reguarding that disease. To educate the patient , nuses should be aware of his educational and social and mental background.

Minimizing the spreading of diseases of a unit is also mostly depending on the nursing staff of that particular unit. To do it they should be aware of new teqniques and should intrdused those and practice those. And they have the responsibility of educating other team members about such methods.

Apart from that a nurse has a great responsibility to prevent the socity they live from decises. It is mostly goes to the public health nurses. They have a great knowledge about every individual In there areas. They should educate the society members of preventive methods. According to each persons health details, family background and education, the public health nurse should recognize the risk factors and should give solutions accordingly. Immunization program also one of the most important program. Nurse is a very important person in this program. The nurse should make sure every member of the society gets involves in this program and should teach them about the importance of this.

Keeping record about what is going on and reporting the authority of particular incidents is also important. Keepiin a eye about epidemic is also important. And in epidemics nurse should educate the society members about how to prevent it.

A particular attention about old people and children should pay. They are easily vulnerable for any thing. Children are the future of a nation. So keeping an eye about there health is a must. Apart from keeping children from physical diseases, nurse must pay attention about there nutrition and mental health. Mental well being is also a part of health for all. From the pregnancy of a mother, the nurse should pay attention about a child's health status. Teaching mothers about breast feeding and the importance of breastfeeding is a key responsibility of a nurse.

Ageing population is also a big problem in future world. There physical and mental well-being is also vital. Regarding this a nurse can do a lot of things. Nurse should guide persons to medical cheek ups regularly. That way risk factors are identified early and preventing them is easy. Old people are easily vulanarable to mental inbalance. To prevent this happen nurse should do something to secure the social status they had. The most important thing is making sure theyget the family support.

Conclusion

I realized the importance of WHO's two most effective concepts about peoples well-being, health for all and primary health care. I also realized the role of a nurse in these concepts and how close these concepts with nursing practice. I understood to get a better approach for an effective nursing care; a nurse must study these concepts closely because most of the nursing practices are based on primary health care and health for all concept.

Apart from that I understood there are other methods of medicine practices and they are also very live. Those methods have advantage and dis advantages. But most importantly still vitally recognized among society as effective methods.